Short Workouts for Beginners

Get Healthier and Stronger at Home

Book 1 in the Jade Mountain Workout Series

By Whit McClendon

Copyrights

Short Workouts for Beginners

Get Healthier and Stronger at Home

Book 1 in the Jade Mountain Workout Series

Copyright © 2016 by Whit McClendon

Cover Art by: lauria
Published by: Jade Mountain Martial Arts, Inc./Rolling Scroll Publishing, Katy, TX
Website: www.jmma.org

Acknowledgements

I've been learning and teaching martial arts and fitness concepts for over 30 years. Not only has it been exceedingly fun for me, but I've taken great pleasure in teaching others to enjoy the benefits of martial arts and fitness training. It has been deeply gratifying to hear back from students, even years later, thanking me for helping them get started on the path to a healthier lifestyle. As much as I've taught my many students, they have also taught me quite a bit. I've had some fabulous teachers both in martial arts and in the fitness industry, so I'd like to thank everyone who has ever spent time on the mats with me in any capacity. Without knowing it, you changed my life.

Brian Briscoe, thanks for inspiring me to write this book. I hope that it can help folks to improve their health and their lives in even a small way.

~Whit McClendon - 2016

Dedication

This book is dedicated to the people out there who are sick and tired of being sick and tired, and are willing to do something about it! I've met and worked with hundreds of folks who want to get in better physical shape but are nervous about getting started because they either don't know what to do or they think that they'll have to kill themselves to get fit. My heart has always gone out to people like that, and I want to help. If this little book can help even a single person to start exercising and live a healthier life, I will have succeeded.

Contents

Introduction 1

Chapter 1 – Getting Started 5

Chapter 2 – Mindset 10

Chapter 3 – Exercises 14

Chapter 4 – Warm Ups & Workouts .. 35

Chapter 5 – Running and Walking 47

Chapter 6 – Summing It Up 54

Afterword 56

About The Author 57

Introduction

If you're reading this book, then it's likely that you want to get healthier and stronger. Congratulations! That spark of desire, that knowing that you want to achieve something beyond what you have now, is a big first step!

After that realization, many folks can be confused as to what to do next. There are a million ways to 'get in shape,' but which one is right for you?

This book is geared towards beginners who want to exercise but need a plan. I've compiled a handful of simple workouts that can be done in the privacy of your own home with a minimum of equipment, often none at all. The workouts are short, as challenging as you want to make them, and very effective when done properly.

I own and run Jade Mountain Martial Arts, Inc, in Katy, Texas, and I work with lots of folks of all ages. Many want to learn martial arts, but others are more concerned with improving their fitness level and their health. In talking with so many of them over the years, I noticed some things that seemed to keep popping up often when we talked about the process of exercising and working out.

The biggest complaint/excuse that I hear when people are giving me all the reasons why they can't exercise is that of time. "I don't have time to get in shape!" I hear it often. However, you truly can exercise effectively without spending a couple of hours to do it, you just have to know how.

When many people think about 'getting in shape,' they imagine getting in their car, driving to a gym, spending at least an hour (more likely two) trying to figure out what weights to lift and then waiting for the machine/bench/weights to be available, getting exhausted, then driving home at last to collapse on the couch. Sound familiar? I thought so. However, I have good news for you! You can get a good workout done in the privacy of your own home in 20 minutes or less. Seriously. Of course, some workouts can take longer, but if you're just starting out and learning your way around this whole 'working out' stuff, then even 15 minutes will likely be sufficient for the time being.

Another thing that discourages many folks is the media. We're bombarded by images on tv and the internet that tell us that guys need to have totally ripped abs, rippling pecs, and bulging biceps to be considered 'in shape,' and girls need to be slender supermodels with zero fat percentage. Well, that's just not true. The main thing you should be concerned with is HOW YOU FEEL. Our students who follow the guidelines in this book consistently report that they feel better and stronger, are sick less, and end up having to buy new clothes because their old ones are too big! They play with their children more, they get more done around the house and at work, and they just feel better. That's certainly worth spending a little time each day to get sweaty!

Improving your fitness and health is an attainable goal. I wrote this book in the hopes that it would illustrate that fact, and help those who just need a little guidance so that they can get started. So read on! I truly hope that it helps you.

Chapter 1 – Getting Started

So you're ready to work out! Awesome!
I'm so glad you've made the decision to
change your life for the better! There are a
few things I'd like to suggest before you move
any further along the path just to make sure
that you're ready for action.

1. **Get a checkup.** If you've been
   sedentary for a while, it is a good idea
   to go see your doctor. Let them know
   that you're going to start a workout
   program. Hopefully, they'll give you
   the go-ahead and you can get right to
   work!

2. **Get some sleep.** Hey, if you're
   doing regular workouts, you're now an
   athlete! Your hard-working body is
   going to need proper sleep so that it
   can rebuild itself into the one you
   want. Make sure that you allot
   enough time each night (or day, if

your schedule works that way) so that you can get 7-9 hours of sleep if at all possible. You'll be more alert, and your body will function far better than it would if you were sleep-deprived.

3. **Drink more water!** Most folks I've met and trained are chronically dehydrated, whether they know it or not. The human body is made up of around 65% water...not coffee, juice, or soda. A mere 5% drop in your body's water level can bring about a whopping 30% drop in your work capacity and mental sharpness! Whoa! It's the kind of thing we all get used to and don't notice the difference until we change it. Yes, you'll go to the bathroom more until your body adjusts, but drinking between 2-3 liters of water a day will help your body become vastly healthier.

4. **Eat the right stuff and avoid the junk.** There are lots of books out

there on proper nutrition and hundreds of different approaches to healthy eating. I suggest that you just keep it simple. Eating lean meats and fish, fruits, and vegetables is a good plan. Go easy on the pasta and rice, but that's generally ok too. Eat regular meals and watch your portions. Avoid like the plague anything that you buy from a drive-through, drink water instead of soda, and maybe save the ice cream and cake for one day a week. "You can't outwork a bad eating plan," is a saying that I keep in mind often. It takes over 500 burpees to 'work off' a large order of fries.

5. **Set yourself up to succeed.** Get your favorite music ready to go. Have your workout clothes laid out. Make sure that distractions are kept to a minimum. Make sure you've got a clear space in which to train. If you

get everything set up ahead of time, then you can jump right into your workout without getting bogged down in the other stuff. It's awfully easy to let little obstacles trip you up and help you make the bad decision to skip it 'just for today.'

6. **Don't obsess over the scale.** Please remember that although tracking your weight can be helpful, that number has only a little to do with your overall fitness. It's just a numerical representation of your relationship with gravity. That's it. I have plenty of students who have been training for months to have their scale only move a few pounds down...but they had to buy new clothes because the old ones were hanging on them and their bodies felt like they were new again. Focus on doing the work and being consistent, and don't focus on the scale.

7. Take rest days. When you first start exercising, a good schedule is one day of work and then rest the next day. After three workout days, maybe take an extra day off if you need it. Then get back to it! Your body needs rest to recover, so give it the time to do so. I also know of folks who work out almost every single day. I'm one of those, but if I start to feel run-down and unmotivated, I won't hesitate to take a day off. Listen to your body.

OK, now that we've gone over those concepts, we need to cover the most important concept of all when approaching any kind of project or endeavor: what's in your head. The next chapter will discuss getting your mind right so that you can get the full benefit from your workouts!

Chapter 2 – Mindset

Before you start sweating it up, let me mention something that I've found to be extremely important: your mindset.

The way you think about your workout program will make or break you, it really will. The good news is that you can relax…you do not have to start with an Olympic athlete's training routine. You don't have to be Rich Froning or Annie Thorsdotter to improve your health. Instead, simply focus on doing what you can do. Start where you are. You may be surprised at how winded you get at first, but that's ok. Start slowly, see how it goes, and move on from there and keep right on moving.

Many of my students have told me that they worry that they are not working hard enough in the beginning. "I'm getting tired during my workouts, and I'm a little sore the next day, but is that enough?" they ask.

10

"Yep!" That's my answer. If you're too sore to move, you're less likely to want to continue your workouts. Of course you're going to be sore, but I want you to ease into this so you'll continue. If you can keep at it, you'll get stronger. One day, you'll find yourself looking back at these first workouts and realizing that your hardest workout back then is your warmup now!

See what you can do. Be brave, but start slowly. Once you learn how your body responds to your training, you can start to push yourself harder. Eventually, you'll find that being exhausted from a challenging workout is momentary, and you'll end up feeling great for the rest of the day!

Not every workout will be your best workout. Honestly, some days, you'll feel like you're rocking it, and others you just won't. That's to be expected. As long as you're not ill or injured, just focus on getting through your workout as best you can. Stay hydrated, eat right, and rest as needed. The next workout will likely be better! Just be consistent and accept that some days will be lower output, while others will make you feel like a superhero!

As you get started, you might have to do Scaled or Modified versions of some exercises. For example, Burpees are pretty high energy, and the majority of my students end up doing the scaled version at first. This is totally OK. If you have to do modified versions of all the exercises, that's not a problem! Don't get down on yourself at all. If you can barely do a single standard pushup, but you can manage several knee pushups, then you DO those knee pushups! You will get stronger as you consistently train, and one day, you'll switch to standard pushups and I'll give you a big high five! Do what you can for now, and you will get better.

As long as you are determined to get started, do what you can, and hang in there, then you are ready to rock and roll! The next chapter will cover a short list of exercises that will be included in the example workouts. Take some time to go over them before you start so you can focus on getting the work done (rather than figuring out the movements) once the clock starts.

Chapter 3 – Exercises

In this chapter, we're going to go over some fundamental exercises that you'll find in the upcoming workouts. In addition, there will be links to short videos that show exactly how to perform the exercises correctly.

Squats

1. Stand with your feet shoulder-width apart.
2. Hold your arms straight out in front of you, palms down.
3. Bend your knees and lower your upper body until your thighs are at least parallel to the ground, ideally until the crease of your hips is below your knees. Keep your knees directly over your feet, head up, and back straight. Focus on putting all of your weight on your heels.

Squats – cont'd

4. Then straighten your legs until you are standing straight and tall again.

5. Video - Squats and Chair Squats

----------------------------> →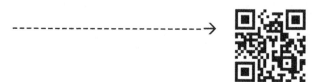

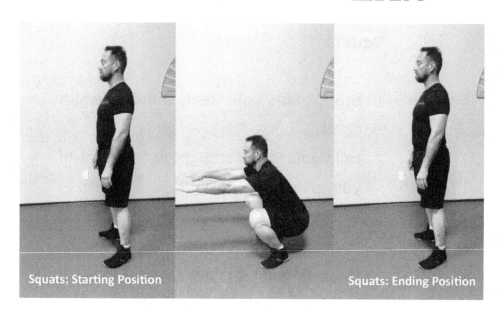

Squats: Starting Position   Squats: Ending Position

Alternate: **Chair Squats**

1. Stand in front of a rigid chair.
2. Lower yourself into a seated position.
3. Stand up again.
4. Video: Squats & Chair Squats

--------→

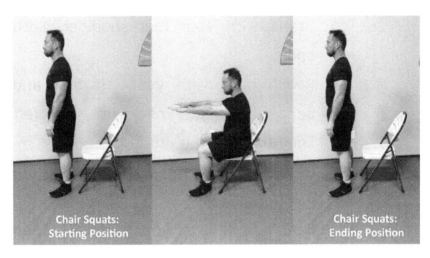

Chair Squats:
Starting Position

Chair Squats:
Ending Position

Lunges

These can be more challenging than squats because you are carrying all of your weight on one leg at a time. Don't be afraid to hold on to a chair or other support if you need help to keep your balance.

1. Stand with your feet shoulder-width apart.
2. Reach back with your left foot and bend your right knee until your left knee touches the ground.
3. Return your left foot to the starting position.
4. Reach back with your right foot and bend your left knee until your right knee touches the ground.
5. Return your right foot to the starting position.
6. Video – Lunges --------→

Lunges – Cont'd

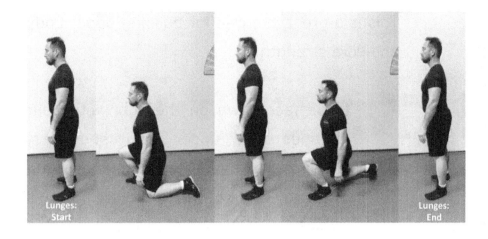

Pushups

This is a great exercise for building upper body and core strength.

1. Lie face-down on the floor with your hands just under your shoulders, palms flat, your feet shoulder-width apart. Curl your toes slightly so you'll be on the balls of your feet when you push.

2. Push down until your arms are completely straight. Keep your body straight (don't sag at your hips). Imagine that your body is a rigid board from your shoulders to your heels.

3. Lower your body back to the start position, or until your chest or belly touches the floor.

4. Video – Pushups and Knee Pushups ---------→

Pushups – Cont'd

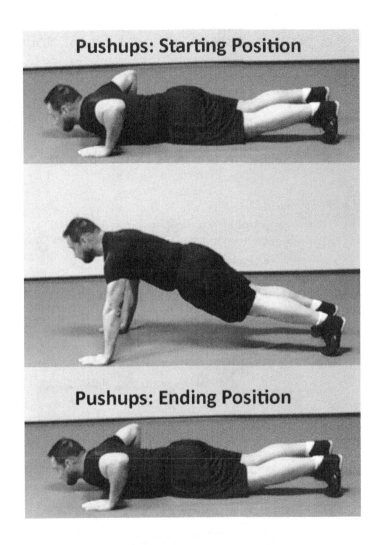

Alternate: **Knee Pushups**

Rest your weight on your knees during the pushup instead of the balls of your feet. Keep your body straight from the shoulder to the knee.   Many folks cross their ankles, but it's not required.

Video – Pushups & Knee Pushups -→

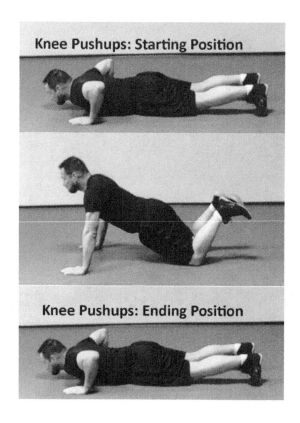

Knee Pushups: Starting Position

Knee Pushups: Ending Position

Alternate: **Wall Pushups**

For some people, Standard and Knee Pushups just aren't workable due to injury or a lack of strength. This variation can help.

1. Stand just beyond arms length away from a wall. Keeping your body straight, stretch out your arms, palms facing out, and lean slightly so that your hands make contact with the wall.
2. Bend your elbows until your upper chest is close to the wall.
3. Straighten your arms and push yourself back to a standing position.
4. Video – Wall Pushups ---→

Wall Pushups – Cont'd

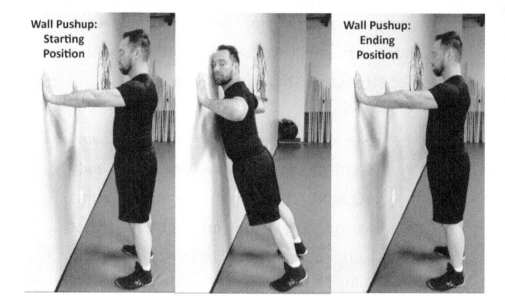

Wall Pushup: Starting Position

Wall Pushup: Ending Position

Sit Ups

An old standard, still a great way to strengthen your abdominal muscles.

1. Lie on your back with your knees up and feet flat. Extend your arms over your head.
2. Bring your arms forward, tighten your stomach muscles, and raise your body towards your knees until you are sitting up.
3. Lower yourself back to a lying position and bring your arms back to where they were.
4. Video – Sit Ups
   and Crunches ------------→

Sit Ups – Cont'd

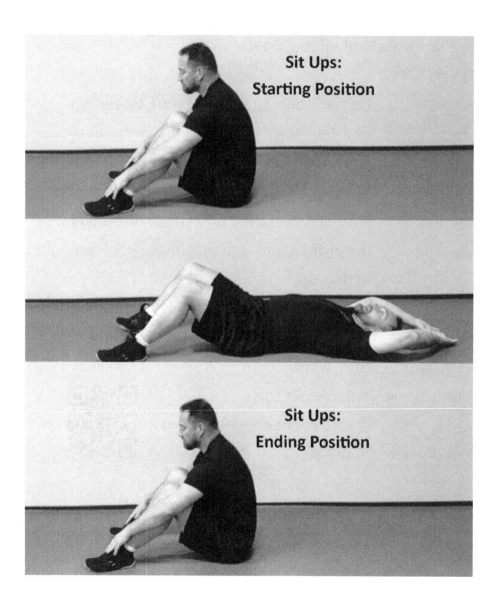

Sit Ups:
Starting Position

Sit Ups:
Ending Position

Alternate: **Crunches**

1. Lie on your back with your knees up and feet flat. Place your fingertips on your head behind your ears, and hold your elbows out to either side.
2. Tighten your stomach muscles, raise your chin, and raise your chest and shoulders up off the ground.
3. Return to your starting position.
4. Video – Sit Ups
   and Crunches ------------→

Crunches – Cont'd

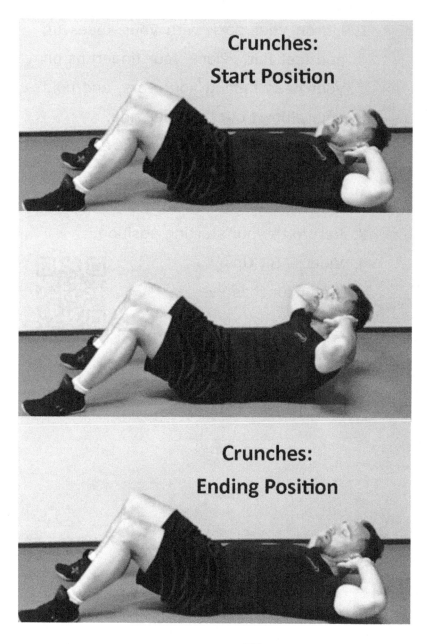

Crunches:
Start Position

Crunches:
Ending Position

Burpees

This is one of my all-time favorites. It's also quite challenging, and your body will definitely get stronger after working with these for a while.

1. Stand with your feet shoulder-width apart, arms by your sides.
2. Bend your knees and squat so you can put your hands on the floor in front of you.
3. Kick both feet behind you into a pushup position and lower your chest all the way to the floor.
4. Straighten your arms (do a pushup) and jump both feet forward so you're back in a squatting position.
5. Jump up and raise your arms overhead.
6. Video – Burpees
   and Scaled Burpees ------→

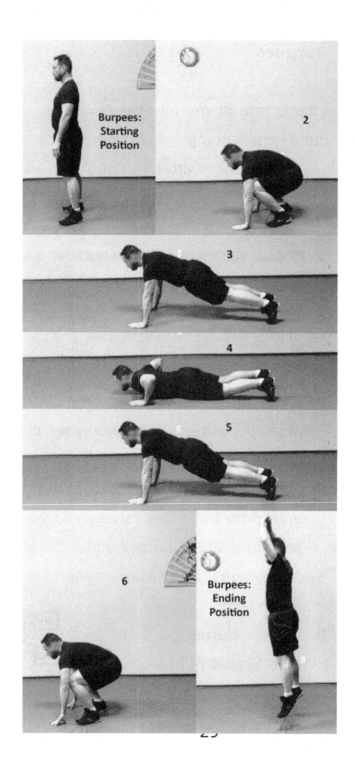

Burpees:
Starting
Position

2

3

4

5

6

Burpees:
Ending
Position

Alternate: **Scaled Burpees**

For a lot of my students, Scaled Burpees are the way to go until they work up to the full version.   A great (and often more doable) exercise.

1. Stand with your feet shoulder-width apart, arms by your sides.
2. Bend your knees and squat so you can put your hands on the floor in front of you.
3. Step one foot back into pushup position, then the other. Drop to your knees if necessary.
4. Lower your chest to the ground, then straighten your arms (do a pushup).
5. Step one foot forward, then the other so you're back in a squatting position.
6. Stand up (no jump necessary) and raise your arms overhead.
7. Video – Burpees
   and Scaled Burpees ------→

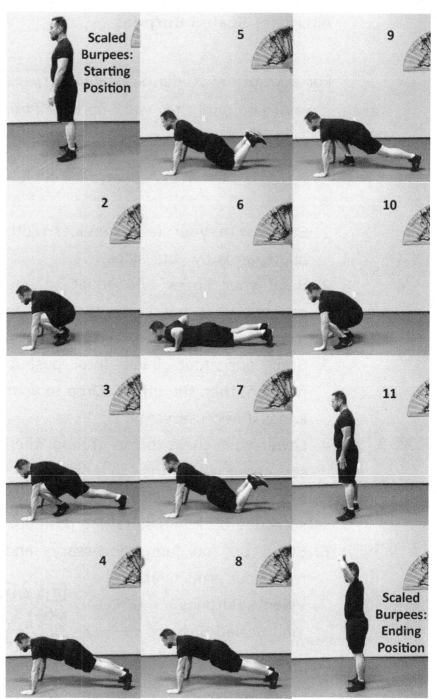

Jumping Jacks

Most folks are familiar with this one, but it's deceptively simple. Do enough of these and you'll be huffing and puffing!

1. Stand with your feet together, arms by your sides.
2. In one motion, jump your feet out to your sides, and raise your arms overhead, touching fingertips.
3. Return to the start.
4. Video – Jumping Jacks ------→

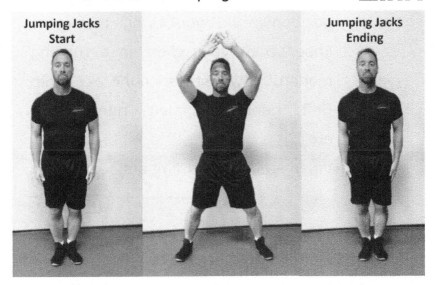

Jumping Jacks Start

Jumping Jacks Ending

Mountain Climbers

These are great for building your cardio capacity and core strength. You'll see.

1. Assume a plank position on the ground, palms flat, arms extended, legs straight. It's the top of your pushup position. Keep your body as straight as possible.
2. Bring one knee towards your chest, then return that leg to its starting position while you bring the other knee up to your chest in a running motion. Two steps count as 1 rep (left, right, ONE, left, right, TWO, etc.)
3. Video – Mountain Climbers

   ------------→

Mountain Climbers – Cont'd

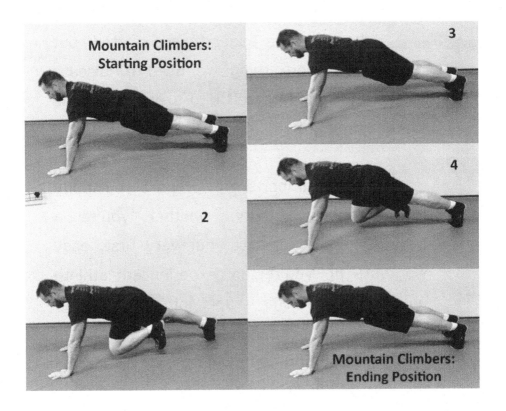

Mountain Climbers:
Starting Position

3

2

4

Mountain Climbers:
Ending Position

Chapter 4 – Warm Ups & Workouts

I know you're eager to get started, but there's one more thing we need to discuss before you fling yourself into a workout: the Warm Up!

It's very important to prepare your body for strenuous activity, whether you're a beginner about to start your very first, easy workout, or you're an experienced athlete about to do some super-intense training. Either way, it's necessary to raise your body temperature and go through a series of motions to 'wake up' your body before you train. I often suggest a very easy jog for those who are comfortable running, but if you're new to all of this, you will want a simple series of movements you can do right there in your workout area before you start.

Oiling the Joints

At Jade Mountain Martial Arts, we have a short set of exercises that we often perform to get our bodies ready to train. We call it "Oiling the Joints." By moving our joints through their range of motion, synovial fluid is pumped into the joints. This lubricates and protects them for more rigorous motions. Our pattern starts at the top of the body and works downwards from there.

Neck: Gently turn your head left and right (as if you're saying 'no') 6 or 8 times. Next, tilt your head back and forth 6 or 8 times (as if you're saying 'yes'). Then tilt it side to side a few times (think of a dog when it hears a funny sound). Last, gently roll it to one side, then to the other.

Shoulders: Roll your shoulders forward a few times, then backwards. Next, twist one arm until your palm faces up, then turn and twist the other arm the same way. (We call it

The Egyptian, after the old pictures in the pyramids) Repeat a few times on each side.

Waist: Letting your arms swing, twist your body to the left, then to the right. Repeat 5 or 10 times. Next, rotate your body as if you had a big Hula Hoop, first in one direction a few times, then the other.

Knees: Keep your knees together, and rotate them first one direction a few times, then repeat in the other direction.

Ankles: Trace the outline of one foot on the floor, keeping your knee still. Move first in one direction, then the other. Then repeat with the other foot.

Video – Oiling the Joints ---→

Now that you've Oiled the Joints, it's a good idea to do a few repetitions of the exercises that you'll be using in whatever workout you choose. Just a few repetitions of each exercise will suffice, then you can get started.

Types of Workouts

There are a few different types of workouts we'll cover in this next section, so let's get to them.

AMRAP

This stands for **A**s **M**any **R**ounds (or **R**epetitions) **A**s **P**ossible. I love running workouts like these because they allow people of very different fitness levels to train simultaneously and everyone gets a great workout! Some super-fit folks might do 15 rounds of work while newer folks might only get 5, but in an AMRAP, everyone gets an opportunity to get a workout that's right for them. Don't worry about keeping up with anyone else, just do what you can do!

X Rounds For Time (RFT)

This stands for a set amount of work that you will try to accomplish. Some folks will complete a workout of 5 rounds of several exercises in just a few minutes, while others take much longer. Either way, you just do what you can do and take note of the time it took you to do it. Remember, the only person you're competing against is the "old you" who didn't work out! Whatever your time is, mark it down, be proud of it, and strive to improve next time.

Circuit

A Circuit is a workout in which you will be doing several different exercises. Starting with one exercise, you will do as many repetitions of that exercises as you can for a set amount of time. Then you switch to the next exercise, and do the same thing. As each time interval passes, you move to the next exercise until you have performed all of the

39

exercises in the workout. That is one round. You can do as many rounds as you decide, or however many the workout calls for.

A Word of Caution!!

I've mentioned that many folks have a tendency to work too hard their first time out. It takes time to get to know what your body can do, especially if you're not an experienced athlete. Or maybe you once were very athletic, but life got busy and suddenly your athletic days are 15 years behind you, but you still feel like you should be able to work out now like you did then. **Don't overdo it!** If you feel sharp pains in any of your joints or muscles, or if you start seeing pretty little sparkles in front of your eyes, **STOP!** This is a process. It takes time to get your body used to working out, so remember that it's OK to take it easy in the beginning!

Now that we've discussed safety and the different types of workouts, let's get started!

WORKOUTS

1. 4 Tens (AMRAP) – 10 minutes

10 Squats
10 Situps
10 Pushups
10 Burpees

Do 10 of each exercise, then move to the next exercise until you've done all four, then start another round. Keep track of how many total rounds you complete, plus how many reps into the final round.

2.   Burpees and Situps, Oh My! (RFT) – 5 rounds

15 Burpees
15 Situps

Keep track of how long it takes you to get through this one. Complete all the reps if you can, whether standard or scaled. Rest as little as possible, but as much as you need to.

3. Jumping Jacks, Pushups, & Squats (Circuit) – 5 rounds

Jumping Jacks	30 seconds
Pushups	30 seconds
Squats	30 seconds
REST	30 seconds

Keep a close eye on your timer for this one. Transition as quickly as you can in between exercises, and enjoy the rest period!

4. On The Floor (AMRAP) – 10-15 Minutes

10 Mountain Climbers
10 Pushups
10 Mountain Climbers
10 Situps

Decide on either 10 of 15 minutes, then start the clock. Note how many times you can get through the series.

5. Legs, Legs, and Jacks (Circuit) – 4 rounds

> 30 Lunges (15 on each leg)
> 30 Squats
> 30 Jumping Jacks

Keep track of how long it takes you to get through this one. Complete all the reps if you can. Rest as little as possible, but as much as you need to.

6. 100 Burpees for Time! – 1 round

> 100 Burpees

This is a very simple workout that we do at my school, Jade Mountain Martial Arts, as a benchmark. Just start the clock and time yourself...how long does it take you to get through all 100? This is a challenge, both physically and mentally. The first time a student completes the workout, it's cause for a celebration! It's not easy! Whether it takes you 30 minutes or 5, it's a big deal to have simply done all 100 Burpees.

7. More Jacks and Stuff (RFT) – 5 rounds

> 20 Jumping Jacks
> 5 Burpees
> 20 Jumping Jacks
> 10 Situps
> 20 Jumping Jacks
> 15 Squats

Run through the sequence 5 times, note your time at the end. I've found that it's helpful to lay 5 coins on the floor nearby so that I can slide one out of line each time I complete a round. It seems easy to keep track of only 5 rounds, but I've had enough folks tell me that using coins to count makes it MUCH easier. Losing track of your rounds during such a workout can be frustrating!

8. Deck of Doom (or Victory...be positive!) (RFT) – 1 round

Another one of our JMMA favorites, but it can take a little longer. For this workout, you'll need an ordinary deck of playing cards. Shuffle them well! Assign a specific exercise to each suit. One of our most popular and easy-to-remember configurations is listed below.

Hearts	-	Burpees
Diamonds	-	Pushups
Spades	-	Squats
Clubs	-	Sit Ups

The number on the card tells you how many reps of each exercise to do. Face cards count as 10 repetitions. The Aces can be either 1 rep or (if you're feeling sturdy) 11 reps. Jokers can either be discarded or Wild! Pick another exercise such as 50 Jumping Jacks or if you have the available space, a short sprint! Turn the first card over, do the designated number of reps for that exercise, then go to the next card.

In the beginning, just try to get through all the cards. It might take a while! As you get stronger, you can use a stopwatch to time yourself as you work your way through the deck. This is a workout that can be an old standby with the exercises listed above, or you can use any four exercises you choose. And with a good shuffle, the workout changes every time!

These are all basic workouts that don't require any equipment other than the space necessary to perform the exercises, a timer or watch, and maybe a deck of ordinary playing cards. Of course, there are many additional things you can to do build strength and burn off your excess baggage, but I wanted to keep things simple in this book. In upcoming books, I'll discuss how to use kettlebells, dumbbells, barbells, jump ropes, medicine balls, and other tools that can help you to get stronger, increase your stamina, and improve your overall health.

Chapter 5 – Running and Walking

Running and walking are two very simple ways of working out to improve your health. This is not to say that they are easy! However, they are generally simpler to get started, don't require a lot of equipment, and there are no complicated movements to learn.

Depending on your current fitness level, you might be able to endure a strenuous run, or maybe walking is the most you can do. Hey, that's ok. Even a brisk walk can get you on your way to better health! First, I'll give you some suggestions to keep in mind before you get started, then a few workouts.

1. **Get good shoes!** They don't have to be the most expensive in the store, but good running shoes should feel great immediately. Don't be afraid to ask for help.
2. **Dress appropriately.** Take the weather into account.

3. **Stay hydrated**, but don't chug before you run. You should be drinking more water all during the day.

4. **Be safe!** Plan your route. Lots of parks have exercise trails, and many schools have tracks you can use after school hours. Keep your eyes and ears open (don't blast your music so loud that you don't hear that truck coming!).

5. **Don't try to set a record the first time out!** This is important. I always tell my new students "Do less than you think you should at first," so that they don't overdo it. In almost every case, those that follow that advice get a good workout, don't hurt themselves, and are ready to train again the next day and maybe push just a bit harder. That's how you start!

Ok, here are a few basic running workouts you can try.

#1 – 10 or 20 Minute Run/Walk

This one is simple. Using your watch or smartphone, set a timer for the amount of time you want to run. Let's say 10 minutes to start. 3...2...1..Go! Run or jog at a manageable speed for as long as you can, then walk when you need to. When you're able, run some more. Keep that pattern up until your time runs out and see how far you've gone. That's it...simple! If you're not up to running or jogging, then just walk instead. If you need to take a break, then take it. The goal is to move continuously for the entire interval. If you can walk the whole thing, then add in some jogging. When you can jog or run for the entire time, then try to do it faster!

#2 – 30 Second Intervals

This one will require you to use your watch or smartphone again. I have an app on my phone that allows me to set up interval workouts, or you could just use a wristwatch that has a countdown timer function. Either way, set yourself up for 30 second intervals.

Run for 30 seconds, then walk for 30 seconds. That's 1 round.

Repeat for a total of 10 to 20 rounds.

At first, just do what you can. Jog, then walk. After working out for a few weeks, you may find that you're able to pick up your speed to a faster run. In time, you can work up to a full-speed sprint! And no, you don't have to keep up with Usain Bolt; I'm much more of a dump truck than a race car. My top speed won't win many races, but it doesn't have to. It's the effort that you're putting out that's important, not the actual speed.

#3 – Running for Distance

Using maps, apps, or the internet, plot a course with a known distance, then time how long it takes for you to cover that distance. Jot that time down, then the next time you run that distance, you can try to go faster. Some suggestions:

½ mile (800m) – 2 laps around an official high school/college track.

1 mile (1600m) – 4 laps

2 miles (3200m) – 8 laps

Whether you run the whole way, walk it instead, or a combination of both, this is a great way to keep track of your progress.

#4 - Couch-To-5K (C25K)

There are quite a few Couch-To-5K apps and programs out there. They can be a huge help in getting started if you don't know what else to do. The programs are meant to help someone who has not done a running program eventually work up to running a full 5K (3.1 miles) without stopping. This can be a great goal since there are lots of 5K fun runs and races in most communities. Get together with friends and start a program together with the goal of participating in an upcoming race...that can be a whole lot of fun!

There are tons of running workouts you can do, including intervals, long distance, and short sprints. Here, I've just provided a few for you to use as you get started. I've known several folks who never ran a day in their lives until they were in their 30's and 40's. Some of them fell in love with running and ended up running half- and full marathons just for fun. This is not to say that you should do that, but who knows? You might find that running is 'your thing,' and do better than you ever before thought possible!

Chapter 6 – Summing It Up

There are lots of ways to 'work out.' Here, I've provided a few simple methods that have helped many of my students improve their fitness level. Try some of the workouts, and see how you do. Then try them again. Be consistent, try to fit in two to four workouts a week for six to eight weeks. Clean up your eating a bit, and drink more water. You'll be surprised at the progress you can make in that time. If you stick with it, you'll end up stronger, fitter, and healthier, with a better quality of life. It'll be worth it.

1. **Start out easy.**
2. **Schedule workouts ahead of time.**
3. **Clean up your eating.**
4. **Drink more water.**
5. **Take rest days!**
6. **Just keep at it. Be determined, and do your best!**
7. **Ask for help when you need it. (I'm just an email away!)**

Follow these steps, and watch your health improve! I hope that this book gives you a nudge in the right direction. Whatever you choose to do to exercise, I hope that you end up happier and healthier!

Afterword

There you have it: details on a handful of effective exercises and a few solid workouts that can help you improve your fitness and overall health. There is no "magic bullet," no single magical program or pill that can give you a rock-hard body in six weeks. It takes effort. That said, the good news is that you have the power to get started, to take action, to start on the path towards a healthier, fitter, and happier YOU. Is it a challenge? Yes. But is it something that you can actually do? YES!! Don't be scared away because you think that it will be too hard or that it will take too long. The time will pass whether you do something or not...so choose to do something that will help you live a better, healthier life.

The End

About The Author

Sifu Whit McClendon was born on October 31, 1969 in Freeport, Tx. He grew up in Angleton Texas and was active in martial arts, track and field, and playing the clarinet in band. After working in the petrochemical field as a CAD drafter for many years, Whit finally realized his life's dream of becoming a full-time martial arts instructor. He now lives with his family in Katy, Texas, plays lacrosse as often as possible, and runs Jade Mountain Martial Arts.

Whit has intensively studied Kung Fu, Krav Maga, Taiji, Kickboxing, and Brazilian Jiu Jitsu since 1982. He has been a CrossFit Lvl 1 certified Coach, a level 2 Kettlebell instructor, and is well-versed in the techniques and applications of cardio & resistance training. He is a CrossFit Games competitor, a 2 time National AAU Shuai Jiao silver medalist, a Tough Mudder enthusiast, lacrosse player, and a 4 time Houston Half-Marathon Finisher.

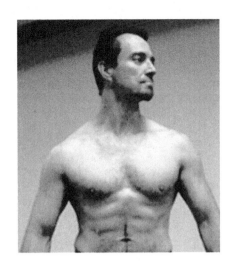

whitmcc@jmma.org

www.jmma.org

www.whitmcclendon.com

Made in the USA
Coppell, TX
22 June 2020